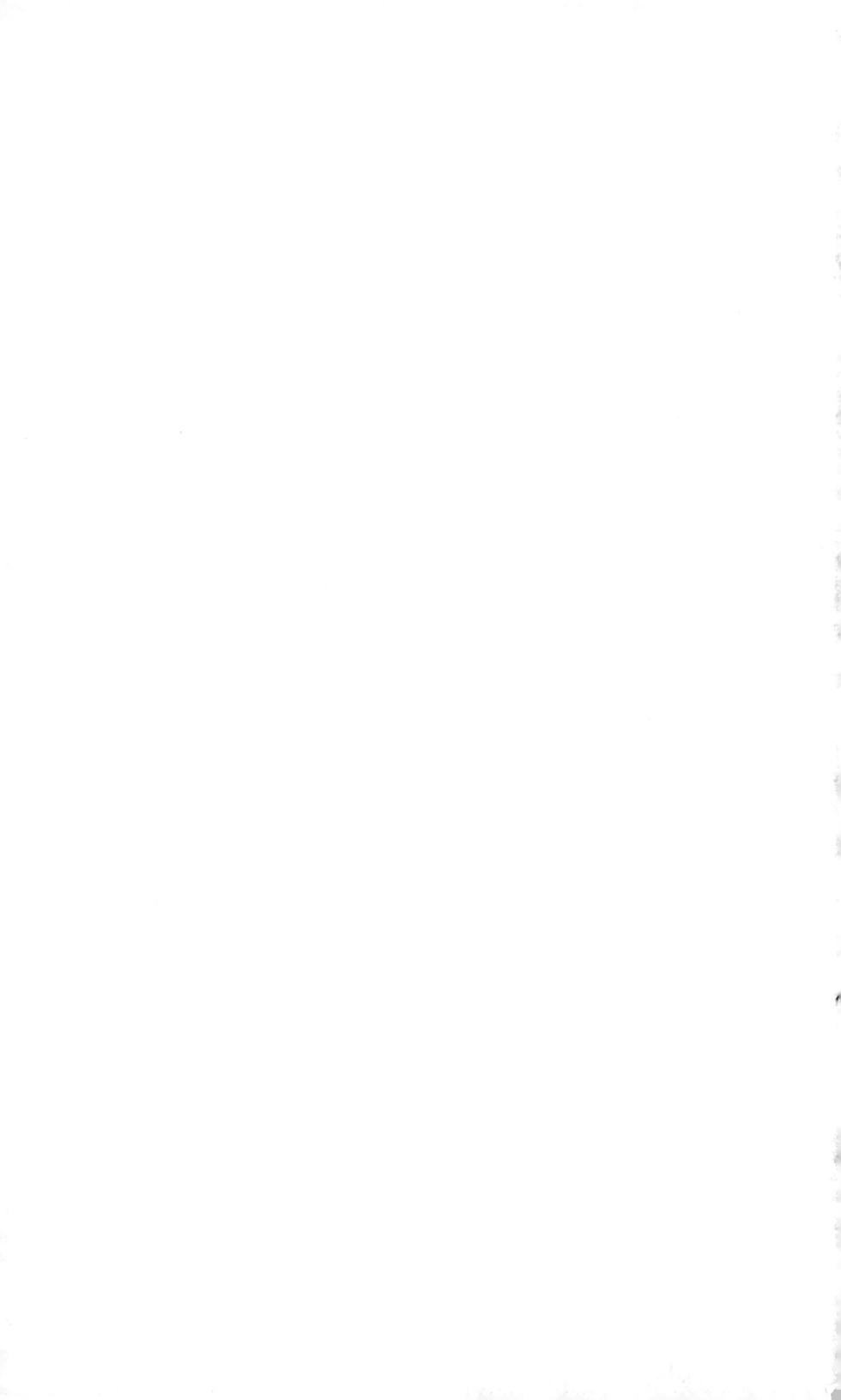

EVERY DAY, ONE DAY YOUNGER

TINA WOODLEY

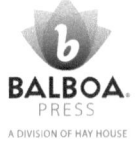

BALBOA.
PRESS
A DIVISION OF HAY HOUSE

Balboa Press books may be ordered through booksellers or by contacting:

Balboa Press
A Division of Hay House
1663 Liberty Drive
Bloomington, IN 47403
www.balboapress.com
1 (877) 407-4847

Print information available on the last page.

ISBN: 978-1-5043-5138-6 (sc)
ISBN: 978-1-5043-5139-3 (e)

Library of Congress Control Number: 2016902251

Balboa Press rev. date: 02/25/2016

CONTENTS

INTRODUCTION

The fountain of youth. For many of us, it's a perennial dream; always present, never realized. We spend the better part of our adult years tracking down its elusive lair, never quite realizing that the fountain of youth is *right in front of our very noses.*

I wrote *Every Day, A Day Younger* not for myself, but for you as a guide to turning back the clock. Its principles apply to all stages of this intriguing journey we call "life." After reading *Every Day, A Day Younge*r, you will look younger. You will feel younger. And most importantly, you will finally understand that age is not only a number but a state of mind.

Every Day, A Day Younger goes beyond mere physical fitness. Its approach is entirely holistic, one encompassing aspects of your spiritual, intellectual and emotional health at all levels.

I wrote this book from my own viewpoint; that of a woman over 50. A time which traditionally coincides with "the big change," also known as menopause. Yet I did not feel any of the so-called changes. I waited for those so-called hot flashes to warm me up. They never came.

It is time to see age in a new light. To do so, you must see getting older as simply another life experience; another new beginning. For me, I like to think of myself as ageless. My hair may be getting thinner, but I am not getting any spots on my hands and face like so many woman around me. I'm not more tired than before. If this is what over 50 feels like, then all women should have this experience!

For me, age has always been a question of mind over matter. And as long as I don't mind, what does it matter?

There was, however, one dramatic change. It seems I went to bed one night with a small waist and got up the next morning being 6 to 8 cm large. I have a stomach where there was none before. It took me a whole year to understand what was happening to me. I felt powerless over the hormonal changes taking place. I knew there must be something I could do.

I tried a philosophical approach After all, isn't '50 the new 30?' The fact that I exercised all my life, I did not realize the importance of my active lifestyle and what a big difference it made in adapting to the aging process.

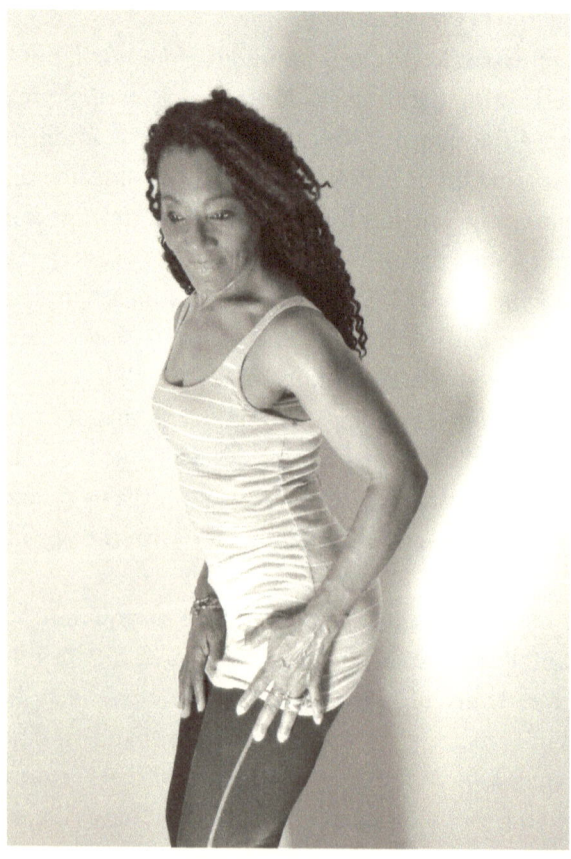

My friends were still telling me how young I looked. People who met me for the first time thought I was 35 - some even thought I was younger. Men younger than my daughter (who is 29) would make passes at me, not knowing I could be their mother.

Thank you sport! Thank you exercise!

Exercise is like the Tin Man's (or woman's) oil can. It can help to counteract many of the negative results of aging, including:

Increased body fat
Decreased bone mass
Diminished strength
Flabby arms and thighs
Muscle and joint stiffness
Impaired balance
Slower metabolism.

If that's not enough, exercise has been proven to preventatively combat the potential for heart attacks, strokes, osteoporosis and diabetes. Nor are the benefits of physical activity isolated to simple physical results; they actually play a significant role in emotional and mental well-being. Simply getting your muscles in motion helps alleviate tension and depression. Neuroscientists have long touted the links between vigorous physical activity and increased serotonin and other forms of "happy" hormones.

If you have not exercised in a while however, please consult your doctor before you begin. A licensed medical professional will be the wisest choice in evaluating the best exercise program for your specific needs. Begin carefully. Do not overexert yourself right at the onset. You may find yourself needing to do aerobic activity up to 30 minutes six times a week or weight training three times a week, but pace yourself. Moderation will prevent overall strain that can damage your body for weeks after injuries (if not longer.)

But exercise is just one part of the story. As I mentioned earlier, I believe in the holistic process, which not only involves diet, exercise and a fundamental understanding of nutrition, but an integral and overall higher awareness of life.

I wrote this book to share my insights on a different approach to your lifestyle, and to present a toolbox for optimal health. If I can change but one person's life as a result, then it's surely been worth it.

In good health,
Tina

PART 1

LIFESTYLE

Chapter 1

AGING AND ATTITUDE

Tool 1: Tap Into Your Inner Fountain of Youth

"I feel like I always have, but I look older. Still, I feel young!" I hear this quite often. Maybe you said it to yourself as a positive statement. After all, it is a good feeling, being young. The problem arises when the way you feel contradicts the way people perceive you.

Other people – particularly in your age group – might see your physical shell and make rapid assessments: "You need to slow down." "Aren't you a grandmother?" "Aren't you too old for that aerobic class?" It might be acceptable to hear that from a younger person; after all, that's still the way they routinely think. Doctors, on the other hand, are notorious for this misconception. So, no matter where you are or whom you're with, hold firm to this truth: "You are as young as you feel."

Tool 2: Learn From Lewis Carroll

In the poem "Father William," a young man asks an older gentleman how he managed to stay so fit despite his age. At first, Father William is patient. But finally, in the last stanza, he gets fed up:

"I have answered three questions, and that is
   enough,"
Said his father. "Don't give yourself airs! Do you
   think I can listen all day to such stuff? Be off,
   or I'll kick you downstairs"

Speaking of poetry, reading and engaging in cultural activities helps keep your mind active and alert. That's why you need Tool 3.

Tool 3: Enrich Your Inner Life

Forget botox. Forget plastic surgery. A rich inner life is the key to eternal youth. Your inner life functions as your anchor, keeping you centered. It helps give you the strength you need to face the outside world. Each and every woman has her own, unique inner life. Some may find it through mysticism and religion. Others choose to become scholars, gaining new knowledge not for ego's sake or professional advancement, but simply to learn all they can about the mysteries of life.

Whatever your circumstances, your inner life belongs to you. Keeping this thought pattern firmly in mind at all times helps keep you young because it leads to an eternal source of vitality, insight, hope and promise. But you need to have confidence!

Tool 4: Find Your Confidence

Concrete confidence is unshakable; however, but a shallow confidence, based solely on physical appearance or what other people think is lost easily. If your confidence is shaky, one key to keep in mind is to "fake it until you make it"; in other words, pretend that it is not. This may be a difficult habit to pick up at first, but if you practice being confident often enough it will become solid, seemingly organic because... that's what it is. Practice makes the master. You will see your life will grow in depth and texture.

Stand up for yourself. Set healthy boundaries and stay true to them. Inside of every woman is a potential warrior. Honor her, acknowledge her and above all respect her!

For example, many of us often hear this: "Well, at your age there are a few things you have to put up with" or "You're looking good for your age". My question then is usually, "Which age is that?" How am I supposed to be looking and at what age? When it comes to your life and your body, ultimately it is your decision. You must take responsibility. You should realize that nobody can give you the right formula to your own happiness (including this book). Let your intuition be the greatest teacher to follow!

If you have been living your life solely to live up to somebody else's expectations, then you need to learn to start doing things your way. And I don't mean the little insignificant things of life. I mean things that really matter. I mean life-changing decisions. Where you live, the work you do, what you eat and your health decisions. Your liveliness, animation, energy and longevity depend upon having the most to say in your life. After all, it's your life to live!

Paradoxically, human beings caught between two opposite needs: solitude and community. It's often difficult to balance the two. Obviously, we as humans need to cooperate: we need to listen to one another, respect other people's opinions and sometimes put our desires aside for the benefit of family or community. But this does not mean refusing to listen to ourselves. Some might call it introversion, while others call it foresight. Whatever you want to call it, it's inside you. Your inner self. It's always there. To give you the answer to the most baffling questions. Never give up listening for it; for it's talking to you, no matter what.

Tool 5: Open Your Mind

Judge Judy has a suitably famous saying: beauty will fade, but dumb lasts forever. People who are set in their ways and closed-minded will never open up to the potential that life offers, and subsequently age quickly. Here are some of the key traits of this type of thinking:

> An attitude of absolute stubbornness - e.g.,"We have always done it this way!"
> Criticizing people who are different or who seem to be expressing themselves too freely.
> An abnormal concern with playing it too safe in all aspects of life.

Developing new habits leaves room for spontaneity. Spontaneity leaves room for serendipity. And serendipity is yet another key to eternal youth. Instead of constantly playing into a constant loop of negative feedback, why not start with some simple affirmations to help keep your mind open to new ideas? Here's a simple game plan:

1) Give new ideas and images a chance.
2) Understand that everyone has his or her own view of truth, regardless of your agreement (or lack thereof!).
3) Remember you can always change your belief, opinion or ideology.

Tool 6: Beauty is a State of Mind: Live By its Rules

1) Embrace the idea of beauty as a state of well-being.
2) Understand the difference between natural, inner beauty and cosmetic beauty
3) Find the beauty in every human being.
4) Celebrate your own beauty by accepting yourself.
5) Never conform to media standards of beauty!
6) Find a definition of beauty that conveys your inner being.

One visible reminder of beauty I suggest is to take the time out to give yourself flowers. Flowers are an energetic life form, putting energy as well as beauty into a room. Give yourself this energy.

As you'll learn in later chapters, you need to start engaging with your personal power house. As a three-time winner of the Ms. Holland title, I learned the importance of beautiful alignment, and a strong, centred stance.

Learn to move beautifully and with grace. One of the most wonderful love songs ever written starts with these words: *"Something in the way she moves/Attracts me like no other lover."* Bad habits, such as slouching or bending forward when you walk, is a sure sign of both poor self esteem and rapid aging.

Tool 7: Choose Friends Who Make You Feel Beautiful

One of the advantages of being an adult is the ability to choose those people whom you call friends. This means you can choose people who see your beauty and acknowledge your value. Those people who see your true beauty are not just people who want to please you, but people who will help you see your beauty and value as well. They ultimately acknowledge you. These are the people who will help you grow younger and wiser.

Tool 8: Meditate and Rejuvenate

Studies have shown that people who meditate on a daily basis have a much younger physiology. Some indicators of physiological aging include:

Short-term memory.
Vision problems.

Increased blood pressure.

Muscle and joint inflexibility.

Meditation helps induce a state of consciousness similar, though not exact, to dreaming or deep sleep. It is surprisingly easy to learn. I have been doing it for years. It's part of the secret to my competition success. Although it takes time and discipline to master meditation, it is one of the best stress reducers I know. Reduced stress sets back the clock in your appearance and your overall health. The lack of stress shows in your face.

Meditation itself can be as simple as sitting comfortably with your back straight (in bed, in a chair, even working in the garden) can be seen as meditation if you are able to keep your focus. It is not a breathing exercise, but a watching exercise. The watching is the meditation. If you have tried meditation before and it did not work, don't give up. Try again beginning with ten minutes a day, or even just five minutes a day.

There is no one way to get to a plateau of focus. If you prefer not to meditate, you can simply sit still with your thoughts or write down your plan for the day. However you choose to relax and find inner peace, try to do it every day at the same time. The regularity of the practice will begin to be second nature.

Tool 9: Listen to Music

Have you been forgetting things lately? Is "Where did I leave my keys?" a constant phrase of yours? Studies have found that listening to music (particularly the style you enjoyed when you were younger) can help! Have you noticed when some people talk about the music of their childhood, their face lights up? This music often bring back memories of their youth At least one person will say, "Wow! That song brings back memories!"

The words "brings back memories" are music (pun intended) to the ears. The results of many studies point to the memory-saving power of music.

Dan Cohen is the founder of Music and Memory—a non-profit organization promoting health benefits associated with music. "A Place for Mom," a facility that treats dementia patients, interviewed Cohen, who gives a unique description of music as being a sort of "back door" which allows the retrieval of forgotten memories. In short, Cohen explains that music helps in restoring brain functionality. Unlike speech and auditory capabilities, which are housed in uniquely specialized regions of the neural map, music prevails throughout the entire brain. This explains why musical memory can be retained even in instances of dementia. Cohen cites a NY State Department of Health study found that people who listened to music for 10 hours a week showed significant improvements in cognitive scores. But as much as we want to keep our memories active, we cannot dwell on negative experiences in the past. That's why we need Tool 10.

Tool 10: Move on and Let Go

Consider this: You must let change happen, and not try to keep things as they are. I know we all want to feel safe, but you cannot navigate life successfully if you are not able to let it go.

If you have had children you will eventually have to let them go off so that they can learn self-growth. If you've held one job for a long time, you may one day be told unexpectedly, "Sorry, the company's closing down." You need to let it go. If you are holding on to anger about something, you need to let it go. If you are angry with your past, you need to find a way to let it out. Most importantly, you need to let it go.

All this letting go doesn't need to happen all at once. You can change your attitude slowly. Start by losing the things that you feel tie you down. You may feel that some souvenirs are worth keeping, but for the most part you can let them go. This may seem like a process of minimization, but in actuality, you're *embracing the essential.* Take a moment to look around your home. How many objects have you been holding on to for years? Objects that you no longer even think about, much less need?

Enjoy the experiences they've brought into your life. But when it's time, you need to let them go. A rule I've learned to live by may sound like a cliche, but if you love someone, they must be set free. Only,in their freedom they will come back to you.

Once you begin understanding that nothing lasts forever - not your job, or your children, sometimes not even your marriage - only then can put yourself in the position of enjoying the changes you make for yourself.

Chapter 2

THE FOUR HEALING
SALVES

In certain shamanic societies, if you came to a shaman or medicine doctor complaining of being disheartened, dispirited, or depressed, they might ask one of four questions.

When did you stop dancing?
When did you stop singing?
When did you stop being enchanted by stories?
When did you stop finding comfort in the sweet
territory of silence?

Tool 11: Dance!

When did you stop dancing?

The birth of Swing Dance coincided with the Great Depression. During this dark era of United States history, some people facing financial ruin chose to jump out of windows and end their lives. Others, despite the gloomy forecast, crowded into the dance halls and danced the night away. Dancing is not just good exercise. It makes you happy. And happy people stay young.

Tool 12: Sing!

Remember your singing days?

In August 2013, Time Magazine published an article entitled "Singing Changes Your Brain." The author noted that singing causes vibrations to move through you, altering your physical and emotional landscape. Group singing is even more powerful. The author equates singing in harmony with mental harmony.

Stacy Horn, author of "Imperfect Harmony: Finding Happiness Singing With Others," notes that group singing stimulates endorphins and serotonin - the same "happiness hormone" that occurs during aerobic exercise! Group singing also releases oxygen, which helps alleviate stress and anxiety.

Tool 13: Read Stories!

When did you stop being enchanted by stories?

Consider the function and power of the narrative of storytelling. Ever since the dawn of history, stories have had the power to enchant, inform, and entertain the minds of listeners, opening doors to wide and seemingly endless possibilities. They allow us a strange ability to experience a range of emotions vicariously, without risking the first-hand turbulence of those emotions. For example, when you cry at the end of a sad book or movie, you experience a release, a catharsis, and not necessarily the trauma that causes it.

Other cultures, their values, their experiences, their histories, their world-views… all spring to life vibrantly through the simple exchange of stories. The history of our ancestors, their trials, our shared human bonds are all illustrated through the sharing of stories. Through the fable, we form a connection with others, realizing our similarities and differences, and encouraging a mutual respect for both. It is the most subtle bond that we can possess. Without it, there is no context. And without context, there is no history.

Tool 14: Take time out for silence.

When did you stop finding comfort in the sweet territory of silence?

"Silence is a source of great strength." ~Lao Tzu

We all need to take time out for peace and quiet. Schedule time to give your brain a rest. No Internet, no TV, no books, no email. One of the reasons why silence is so critical is that it gives us time to go into ourselves and listen to the wisdom that cannot be spoken, but understood only by the heart. Make certain you give yourself enough time to look inwards. Keep an open ear, and you'll eventually hear with the greatest clarity of all.

Chapter 3

TRAVEL

Tool 15: Travel the World

At age 21, I received an invitation to compete in the first powerlifting contest in the USA. Not only did this benefit my career, it introduced me to international travel. As I travelled to different countries, I made new friends, learned about different cultures and helped grow to become the person I am today.

Travel introduces us to new experiences. It opens our mind, gives us a global perspective, and keeps us from getting stuck in our ways. That, in itself, gives you a youthful perspective on life.

Likewise, the trials and tribulations of travel builds confidence, and confidence (as you'll remember from Chapter One) contributes to a youthful demeanor.

A visitor to the Mediterranean or South America just might discover that an afternoon siesta could give them the perfect jolt of rejuvenation if they are used to the more traditionally American habit of working despite exhaustion. In Italy, the "passeggiata," or traditional after dinner walk, encourages both digestion and the burning of fat. These simple traditional customs often have entirely beneficial results because they seem so foreign to our habits and customs, particularly in a day and age in which the 40-hour work week is quickly becoming a 50-60 hour one.

The wider your breadth of experience, the wider your context. The wider your context, the greater the personal growth.

Tool 16 : Redefine Home

Travel helps redefine your definition of the word "home."

After living in many countries, (Bonaire, Holland, Austria and Germany) I realized home is wherever you feel well. For some, this is not an easy decision. In many circumstances, your objectivity and subjectivity will engage in battle.

Here are some examples:

> You want to stay near your birthplace, in order to be near family, but you can no longer tolerate your country's politics.
>
> Your ongoing anger at your government's policies cause stress, and stress destroys your health.
>
> You love the excitement of the big city, but crime, pollution, crowded commutes and corporate competitiveness interfere with your enjoyment. Once again, the stress monster destroys your health.
>
> You have a pre-existing medical condition, and your country's health care policies are extremely expensive.
>
> You love where you live, but rents are so high that you spend hours at work, and never get a chance to enjoy your surroundings.
>
> You move to the high altitude mountains of Colorado, Utah or Europe. At first, the ability to ski and hike works wonders. As you get older, your doctor informs you that the higher elevations are wreaking havoc on your lungs.
>
> Your country of origin does not respect older people.

In these situations, some people just grin and bear it. On the other hand, people who travel know that there are many other alternatives. And while moving to another country is challenging, it's not impossible. In fact, it just might open your eyes.

EXERCISE

Chapter 4

THE FOUNDATIONS
OF FITNESS

As I mentioned in the introduction, exercise like the proverbial Tin Man's oil can from *The Wizard of Oz*. As a tool of rejuvenation, it helps to counteract much of the necessary baggage of growing older. But before you start an exercise program, you need to get back to basics. Let's start with what body trainers call "the powerhouse."

Tool 17: Find Your Powerhouse
and Learn How to Use It

In addition to bad posture, slouching compresses organs and impedes full breathing. That's why you have to constantly remind yourself to stand tall. We frequently do this by lifting out of your solar plexus (just above your navel), and separating your midriff from your lower abdomen. One benefit of this is that it makes your waist look smaller, but it also does something else:

It makes you look powerful!

Nowadays, people refer to this region as "the core." But as a former competitive powerlifter, I believe that Joseph Pilates had a better word:

"The Powerhouse!"

All your movements stem from your Powerhouse. Drawing your belly button toward your spine is similar to pushing the "up" button on the elevator. It empowers the elevator to move up.

Speaking of upward movement, how do you think powerlifters are able to lift so much weight? Yes, they do need strong arms and legs. But they also need strong, toned abdominal muscles: the proverbial six-pack.

It's the deeper core muscles, those closer to the spine, that protect your lower back and keep you balanced during those heavy lifts. And engaging your powerhouse helps improve your posture.

Tool 18: Stand Tall, Strong and Proud

You could instantly appear 12 pounds thinner and years younger anytime you wish. The secret lies in your movement; or perhaps better said, how you carry yourself.

Whether you hold your body straight or you bend forward, your posture will reveal to the world your age In fact, your posture will be a representation of your inner self. If you choose to move gracefully, this will tell the world you are comfortable with who you are. If you choose to hold yourself constrained and timid, this will also be a reflection of your inner state.

A professional will look at your posture and skeletal alignment and be able to predict your injuries, your aging process, your athletic skill and your lifestyle. They can do this because their eyes are trained to notice disturbances and curvatures even from a casual distance.

In traditional villages, women carry vessels of water and fruit on their heads. Ascending the mountains and descending the valleys, they never lose their balance. This would not happen without perfect postural alignment. Just imagine what would happen if these women slouched!

How to Maintain Posture:

Chin is tipped in line with the neck.
Neck is in line with the spine.
Shoulders are back down and relaxed.
Back is straight.
Pelvis in a neutral position.
Knees are neither locked nor bent.

Your body should be relaxed but standing tall. The same applies to posture when seated. Your legs should be at a 90° degree angle when seated.

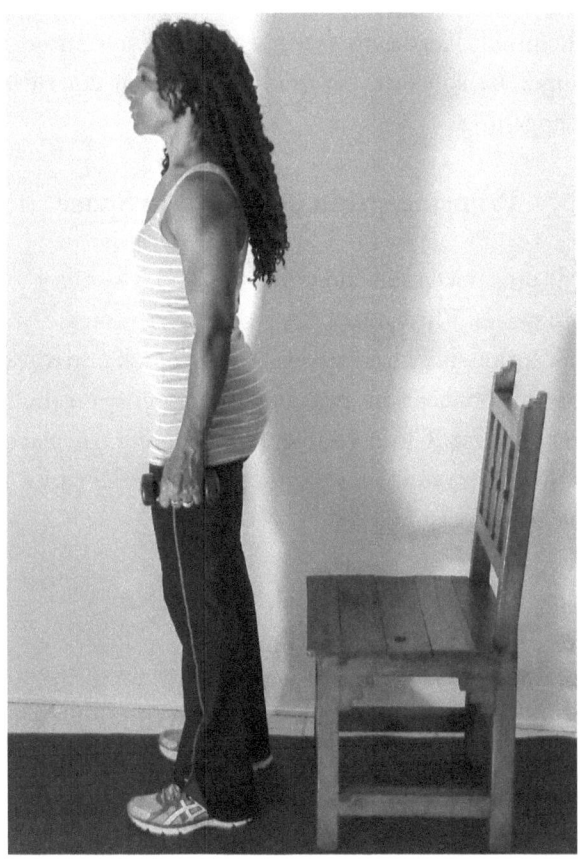

Tool 19: How to improve Your Balance

Life is a balancing act. Every day, we balance our time, our money and our emotions, with hopes of finding equilibrium. Physical balance and emotional balance are similar. Finding your physical center helps you regain your emotional center. Balance is therefore the foundation of physical and mental fitness.

You may ask "why is this important?" Poor balance and proprioception – the sense of how your limbs are balanced – interferes with your ability to perform those exercises correctly.

Most children have incredible balance. They can run, play hopscotch on one foot, and ride a skateboard Balance normally remains excellent throughout the early twenties to the early forties. But in the middle forties to seventies balance starts to deteriorate. The changes are so subtle, so gradual, that you don't ever realize what is happening.

Proprioception or Found in Space

The word "proprioception" describes your body's ability to sense its position in space. When you walk up or down a staircase, you engage in proprioception, because you usually don't look down at the steps.

To test proprioception, place a piece of paper on the floor and stand on top of it. Close your eyes and march in place for one minute. Now open your eyes. If you're close to the paper, you have acceptable proprioception.

Foot and Ankle Exercise

Ankle sprains typically tend to be recurring problems. Once you sprain an ankle, you will probably sprain the same one over and over again. That's because every sprain diminishes ankle proprioception. This foot and ankle training program will help you break this cycle.

Start with a series of 20 heel raises, followed by 20 toe raises. Then, walk forward and backward on your toes, and forward and backward on your heels. Take 10 steps in each direction.

Balance Progressions

If you are a novice, start with single leg balance exercises on a flat surface. When you can hold a position for 30 seconds, try the same movement with your eyes closed. Once you master that hold with your eyes closed, progress to standing on balance training equipment. Start with a two legged balance, then try a two-legged balance with eyes closed. Gradually build up to one-legged eyes open and eyes closed balance exercises. Always have a friend on hand to spot you during these exercises.

Tandem Walking

A narrow base of support increases balance challenge. The tandem walk involves walking across the room, placing the heel of one foot directly in front of the toes of the other. When you complete the forward movement sequence, try the same movement travelling backward.

Hint: Engaging your powerhouse during these exercises will help you keep your balance!

Chapter 5

WHY STRENGTH TRAINING?

You think you don't need strength training? This checklist may prove you wrong:

- Do you notice fat where once there was muscle?
- Are you too tired and worn out at the end of the day to do anything physical?
- Is there a problem with maintaining your weight, even though you're eating less?
- Are you feeling or looking older than you are?

If you have answered "yes" to any of these questions, you may need strength training.

For many women past 35, loss of strength and lack of vigour are painful experiences. If you are experiencing this, you may feel it's an inevitable part of getting older. The main reason most people slow down when they feel older is that they lose about a third of their muscle mass between age 35 and 80. Inactivity plays a major role in the loss of muscle mass.

Have you ever been bedridden for a few days? Do you remember that weak feeling when you try to get up again? Imagine this perpetually, and you'll know what inactivity does to your body.

The first signs are that your legs get tired more quickly, and even a simple act such as standing up from a sofa becomes difficult.

Tool 20: Start a strength-training program

A challenging and progressive strength training program can build muscles and increase strength in women of all ages. Studies have proved that the benefits go even further, including:

Halting bone loss

After menopause, a woman usually loses 1 percent of her bone mass, and sometimes even more during the first five years. She may even develop osteoporosis, a condition in which bones become so porous they easily break. Strength training can help stop the process.

Balance

Our ability to stay in balance also declines over the years. Changes happen so slowly you may not notice it until you are in your seventies. Strength training improves your balancing ability.

Preventing Osteoporosis

Improvement in strength, bone density and balance reduces the risk of serious problems. Should you have osteoporosis, strength training cuts the risk of fractures by improving strength and balance. Women who don't exercise lose up to two percent of their bone density per year.

Many women in fitness studios only do aerobic training and are discouraged from strength training. But if muscles are weak, aerobic exercise will be difficult. After a month or two of strength training aerobic workout will become easier and more fun.

Training muscle also boosts metabolism, supporting weight loss and body toning. Instead of losing muscle, you lose fat because muscle is active tissue. It consumes calories. Stored fat, on the other hand, uses very little energy. When you strength train while following a weight reduction program, fat melts away. When you get rid of fat and build muscle, you can eat more.

Aerobic exercise is essential for cardiovascular fitness. But it won't make you strong. I have seen many aerobic trainers who are flabby and underdeveloped. People often confuse strength training with bodybuilding. Bodybuilding is a sport, which aims to build big muscles, but this is not our goal. Strength training has been the secret for staying slim in Hollywood for ages. To produce big muscles you must train with extremely heavy weights, two or three hours every day, following a very rigorous diet. My strength-training program does not approach those extreme results. This program is to help you increase your strength and from your figure.

Anyone can follow this program. Strength-training principles are the same, regardless of your age or gender. It's really very simple. You work with weights that are just heavy enough so you can lift them eight times in good form before you have to rest. As you get stronger, the weight will no longer challenge you. That's when you need to increase the load and/or the repetitions.

Chapter 6

I WANT MUSCLES

Your body houses more than six hundred muscles. Together, they account for a third of your weight. Muscles drive every move you make.

As children and young adults, women have all the muscular capacity they need. But somewhere in midlife that changes. Starting around age 40, most women lose almost 250 grams of muscle each year, while gaining the same amount of fat. By age 80, they have about a third of the muscle mass they had at forty.

Once you understand the importance of muscle work, you will appreciate the powers of strength training.

Muscle Actions

For every action, there's an equal and opposite reaction. This also applies to your muscles. As one muscle group contracts, the opposing muscles lengthen:

> As your quadriceps contract or shorten, your hamstrings stretch or lengthen.
> As your biceps contract or shorten, your triceps stretch or lengthen.

> As your chest muscles contract or shorten, your
> back muscles stretch or lengthen.

Your muscles perform three types of contractions:

Concentric contractions, the lifting phase of the exercise, shorten the muscles. Eccentric contractions, the return phase of the exercise, lengthen the muscles. Isometric contractions do not change the length of the muscle. However, they are involved in the stabilization process. For example, when you do a biceps curl from a standing place, your deep abdominal muscles contract isometrically, to help stabilize your spine.

All contractions are important. Many people lift a weight, then simply drop it on the return movement. Doing this deprives them of an important factor: the eccentric contraction. Likewise, you can improve the effect by adding an isometric contraction. For example, when you reach the peak of a biceps curl, squeeze your biceps for one second, as if you were showing off your muscles. Then, lower the weight in a slow, controlled movement.

Bone Density

Weight-lifting not only tones your muscles: it can help prevent loss of bone density.

Your body contains over two hundred bones, joined by cartilage and ligaments. When you touch your bones through soft skin, they feel solid but this is just the outer wall. Underneath, your bone tissue is porous and very much alive.

Bone is made of calcium and other minerals; that's why it is hard. Like muscle, bone tissue constantly repairs and renews itself, though more slowly. This process is known as cell remodelling. Osteoporosis breaks down damaged bone, releasing calcium into the blood.

Your bones grow through your entire life, but over the years the balance shifts between building and breaking down. This occurs until the age of 25. From the ages of 25 to 35, you maintain bone density if you're healthy.

Yet, as menopause occurs, you can lose up to one percent of bone density. This loss is natural. During this time and up to five years after, you can slow down the loss through physical activity. Between the ages of 55 to 70, bone loss typically slows down (but you can still lose an average of one percent per year.) At 70 and older, loss slows down even further to less than half a percent a year.

Osteoporosis depends on many factors; some are preventable and some are not. These include:

> *Gender.* The risk is much greater for females.
> *Age.* The older you are, the greater the risk.
> *Race.* The lighter your skin, the higher your risk.
> *Heredity.* If there's a family history, the risk is much higher.
> *Body Type.* The thinner you are, the stronger the risk.
> *Early menopause.* For example, if you reached menopause before age 45.

Prevention is the best cure. And strength training can prevent osteoporosis. It encourages continual muscle and bone renewal. By challenging your bones with weight-bearing exercise, you can help maintain your bone density. It also increases the metabolic rate, helping you maintain your weight. Think about this: one-half pound of muscle loss occurs every year after the age of 25. This produces a one-half percent reduction in basal metabolic rate (BMR) each year. A reduced BMR means that you are less able to use the food you eat as energy. This unused food gets stored as body fat.

Tina Woodley

Re-sculpting the Body Beautiful

Your body starts to change at adolescence. It changes again after childbirth and once again at menopause. Suddenly, your breasts surrender to the forces of gravity, your waist thickens and your belly rounds. Will exercise help? Yes, but be realistic. Accept the fact that you will have a different shape during your 50. Try not to make value judgements. Re-sculpting your body begins with self-acceptance. It means accepting the number of years you have lived in this body and praising yourself for its beauty. It also means changing your eating habits. Your body needs less food as you get older so you cannot eat the same way you did before. Although your metabolism will slow down, regular exercise can keep it from coming to a halt.

Chapter 7

PREPARING FOR A POSITIVE CHANGE

By now, you should realize how important exercise is to maintaining your lifestyle. But in the real world, you may find an enormous gap between preaching and practice. Does any of the following sound familiar?

> *I don't have the time or money for fitness. My knee hurts. My back hurts. My blood pressure is high. I am too old. I am too unfit – I need to get in shape first.*

Depending on where you live, joining a fitness studio can be expensive and time consuming. There are much safer and inexpensive ways for women of any age or fitness level to begin an exercise program. All you need to do is decide when. But, it may be necessary to check with your doctor before starting any physical activity.

Ask yourself the following:

1) Have you ever been told by a doctor you have a history of heart problems?
2) Have you felt any pain in your chest in the past month when doing physical activity?

3) Do you easily lose balance or feel dizzy?
4) Is there a history of joint problems?
5) Are you taking medication for high blood pressure?
6) Is there any reason you know of why you should not do physical activities?

If you answered yes to one or more of the questions above, you should see a doctor before establishing an exercise regimen. If you answered no to all questions, start becoming more physically active. Begin slowly and build up gradually. Your doctor can tell you what type of exercise you can safely perform.

My Story

Many years ago, when I first began strength training, it was exciting to be doing something that other women were not. It made me feel good about myself and, as I got stronger, it soon became part of my identity.

Many women tell me that they are too busy and they don't have time for exercise. But there are many possibilities even if you are one of those busy people.

Exercise before work or during lunch hour. Workout while watching television. Or even get up earlier two mornings a week.

Think positive about the benefits you can gain!

Yes, there are record numbers of fitness studios. But far more people are sitting on the couch or at the computer all day. It is hard to translate knowledge into action. All of us struggle to make positive changes in our lives. In the process, we discover the challenge of rearranging behaviour. Here are five stages you'll pass through as you make strength-training part of your life:

The Preparation Stages

Stage 1 – Precontemplation

You don't have time for exercise. You don't really see the need for it and don't realize what it can do for you.

Stage 2 – Contemplation

You have become interested in fitness training. You know it will make you stronger and healthier, but are waiting for the right moment to begin.

Stage 3 – Preparation

You are not training with weights yet, but you have begun to start walking and plain on making a concrete program.

Stage 4 – Action

You have begun to change your eating habits and feeling better about yourself. The first steps of a strength-training program have become routine.

Stage 5 – Maintenance

This is the stage where strength training has become a habit and you begin to see real benefits to your health and well-being. I have seen women move from habit to an incredible sense of empowerment and spiritual well being. They look younger and feel better than they have for many years. And because of this, their training has become an integral and all-encompassing part of their lives.

Chapter 8

YOUR WORKOUT TOOLS

Don't feel like joining a gym? Or is your budget too cost-prohibitive to allow you to take advantage of the ever-increasing membership rates? Don't fret! In this chapter, I'll tell you how you can create an inexpensive exercise area in your own home. Here's what you'll need:

> Ankle Weights
> Dumbbells
> A sturdy chair
> A towel
> Comfortable clothes

Using free weights

Free weights are weights held in your hand or strapped to your body, in contrast to weights that are part of a machine. This is the least expensive type of strength-training equipment. You can start this program with two types of free weights – ankle weights and dumbbells.

Ankle Weights

The simplest form of ankle weights are strap-on cuffs with a compartment for up to 6 kg. You can adjust the weight of the cuff by adding or removing these bars.

In the beginning, you'll only need to work out with 1 or 2 kg on each foot (depending on your strength.)

Dumbbells

During the first week you will be doing arm exercises with dumbbells weighing 1 - 2 kgs. Dumbbells can be purchased in one-kilo increments from one to 6 kg.

Chair or Ball

Some exercises will be stationary while sitting, while others require standing and holding on to a chair. If you are not certain of the height, experiment with different chairs. Each should be sturdy, armless, and with a seat high enough that you can sit all the way back with your feet barely touching the ground (your knee joints should be just over the edge of the seat.) In addition, it should have a back high enough that you can stand behind it without bending over.

If you use a ball, your knees should be at a 90-degree angle when you are sitting. The ball adds a balance challenge to the exercises, which helps you use your core muscles!

Leg exercises are done seated with a rolled-up towel under your knee, working as a pad to keep them in the correct position.

Chapter 9

THE FIRST 10 EXERCISES

These are ten basic, but effective, exercises. It is important to understand the movement of each one. Start with light weights (perhaps 2 or 3 kgs) for your legs. Once you find your strength and stamina improving in a few short weeks, you'll be able to use more on both arms and legs.

Your training time should be no less than 30 minutes a day. You can do the major muscle groups at the beginning of the week, working from big to small muscles.

EXERCISE 1

Squats

Squats are particularly important for legs in that they not only strengthen them, they help shape them.

The squat is a basic, foundational exercise chiefly because your feet maintain a fixed position. This is what is known as a closed chain exercise, and are ideal for helping to build bone density and prevent osteoporosis.

When performing the squat, it's important that you start by bringing your hips back. Not by bending your knees. Keep your back straight and your spine neutral, your chest and shoulders erect.

As you squat down, focus on keeping your knees in line with your feet.

To build a muscle you should do eight to twelve repetitions. Rest for a few seconds, then repeat the repetitions. You can also encase the weights for each new repetition.

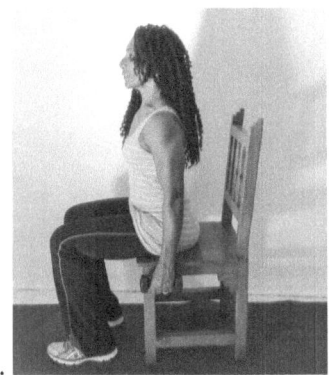
A.

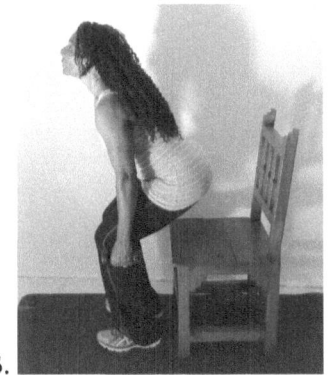
B.

EXERCISE 2
Standing Leg Curl (with ankle weights)

This exercise can strain your hamstrings (found on the back of your legs) when using weights, so be careful to stretch after every workout.

Keep your back straight. Stand behind a chair, bending your legs 24 degrees. Bring your heel to your bottom and *slowly* bring it back to the starting position. Repeat this movement 8 to 12 times, alternating your legs. Aim for three sets.

EXERCISE 3
Leg Extension (with ankle weights)

Known as the quadriceps, this is the most visible leg muscle in front of the thighs.

Keeping your back straight, lift your leg from the knee up and bring it back slowly. Put a towel behind your knee on the edge of the chair as a pad. The movement should be down slowly.

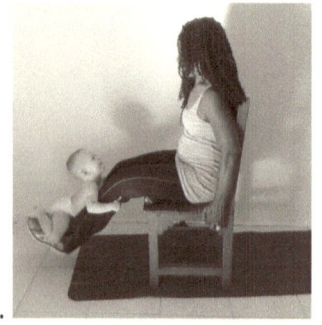

A.

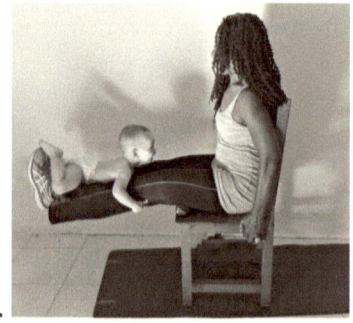

B.

Note: My grandson insisted on getting into the picture, so I used him instead of ankle weights!

EXERCISE 4
Side Leg Raise (with ankle weights)

This exercise helps strengthen and tone the hip abductors, slenderizing the torso.

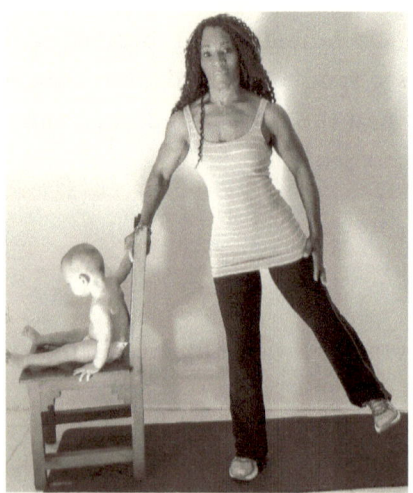

1. Standing in a upright position, lift your leg out to the side of your body and return to the starting position. It is best to hold on to a wall or chair leg. You should be slightly bent, then slowly move the leg away from the body keeping it raised.

EXERCISE 5
Dumbbell Curl

Most women I meet don't like to train their biceps muscles; an unfair judgement, since they assume that they will become appear more masculine. But this muscle plays a huge role in the process of aging. If there is no muscle in the arm, the skin will turn flabby and sag.

Keep your elbows to your side while performing the curl. Move the weight slowly up to shoulder height and back down without bending your wrist.

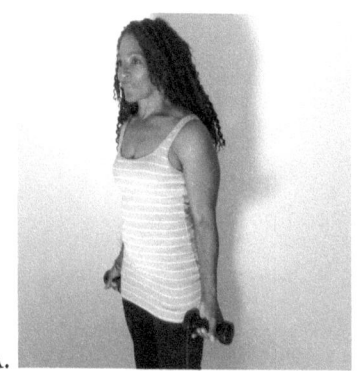 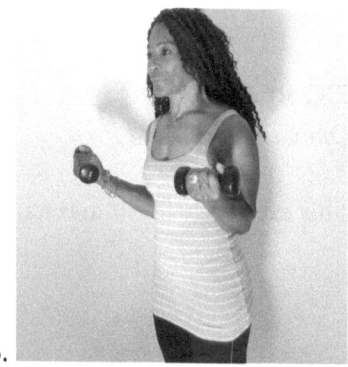

A.   B.

EXERCISE 6
Triceps Extension

This exercise can help alleviate flabby skin hanging on the back of the arm.

Bend forward and keep your back straight and your knees bent. Hold a dumbbell in each hand with your palms facing upwards. Lift and release.

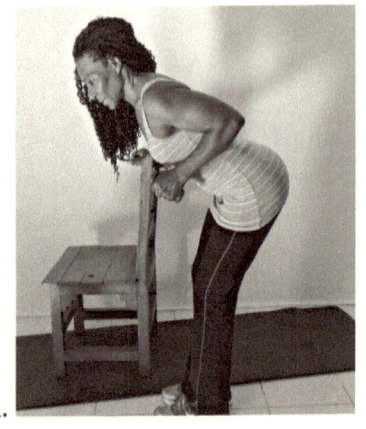 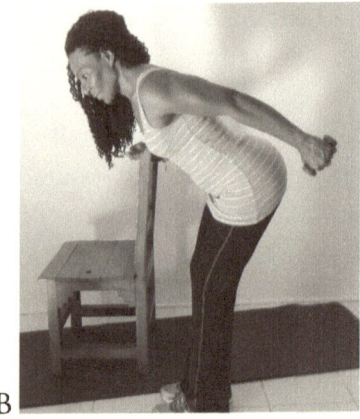

A.   B

EXERCISE 7
Dumbbell Overhead Press

This exercise helps in maintaining good posture.

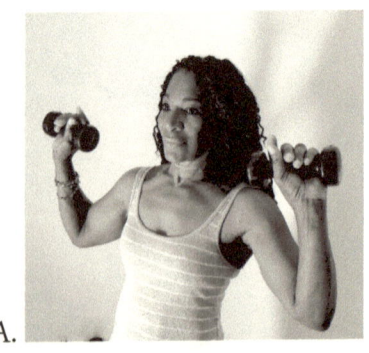 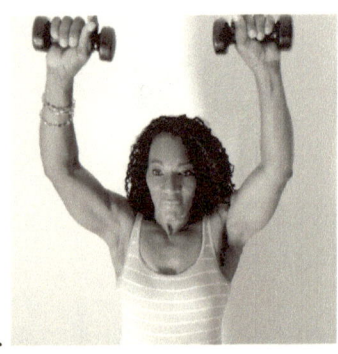

A.   B.

EXERCISE 8
Upright Rowing

This is a perfect exercise to improve both shoulder strength as well as posture. Your hands should be as wide apart as possible. Keeping the inside of your hands facing down, use two dumbbells of equal weight to slowly "row" back and forth.

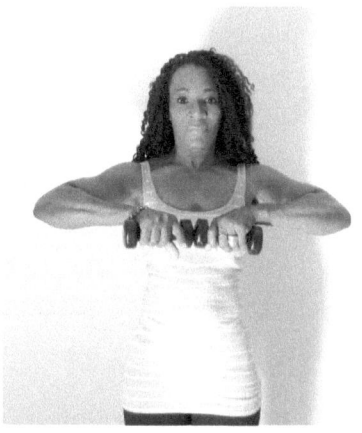

EXERCISE 9
Toe Raise (with or without weights)

This is a simple and effective exercise to straighten your calf muscles and make them more flexible. Each movement should be done slowly.

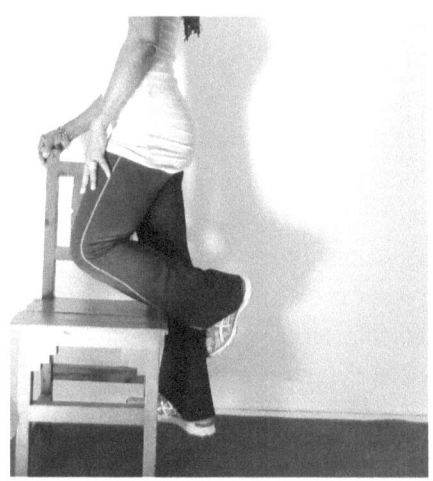

The First Three Months

The first three months of strength training is a special time. You are forming a habit that can and will change your life. During this period, expect interesting improvements. This is the time when change is most rapid.

Month 1. You will learn the exercises using lightweights. Your first session may take longer than an hour, but it will soon seem more efficient. Some women experience minor aches and pains during the first two weeks. But by the end of the first month, the exercises will be familiar, and you will be performing them correctly and with more intention.

Month 2. This is when you start to see and feel results. Some of the exercises may find you lifting twice as much than you did at the beginning. Many women notice that they feel stronger and more energetic. If you were sedentary before, you may notice changes in everyday activities. If you were already fit, improvements may be evident only when you push yourself.

Month 3: You are entering a new and important phase in strength training, when your muscles begin to change. It may seem slow, but fret not; your body has already gone through lots of changes. Your muscle cells are getting bigger, and your bones are starting to react to the stimulus of strength training.

You will feel revitalized after three months of strength training. You will have more energy and move more quickly. Some women may lose weight while others won't, but your body will become more firm and sculpted. The more out of shape you were in the beginning, the more noticeable the improvement.

How long should you continue to exercises? That's up to you. For me, strength training is a lifetime goal.

However, it's best not to use more than 4 kg with ankle weights. Instead, switch to exercises that use your body weight for resistance or strength-training machines for your arms. Don't lift dumbbells that are heavier than 6 kg. Switch to machines for more arm exercise.

You should follow this program for at least 4 to 6 weeks. For one, it takes about four weeks to settle into any program. As you become familiar with the routine and become more adept at the exercises, you'll begin to notice the changes.

After four weeks, you are no longer a beginner. But you need at least eight more weeks - perhaps longer - for your routine to become a habit. If you record your progress in your fitness program, you'll find yourself more likely to continue. Try keeping a record for at least the first twelve weeks. This helps in two ways:

Motivation: These exercises improve your strength and health quickly and acts as an encouragement for even more changes.

Efficiency: Simply put, training goes more smoothly when you keep records.

Training with a friend

Having an exercise partner is the next best thing to hiring a professional trainer. It helps give you the structure and commitment of a regular schedule. You and your partner can check each other's form. And your workouts will be more fun. If one of you hits a low point, the other can provide a boost.

Chapter 10

CREATING AN INDIVIDUAL PROGRAM

So far, you've learned how to perform the exercises. The next step is to turn them into an individualized program and make fitness part of your lifestyle. As you get stronger, training must be more challenging and you will need to adjust your program to meet the challenges. Using the right weights for each exercise is the key to both safety and success.

Where and how to start

The greatest amount of weight you can lift just once is your maximum strength capacity. You will be working out at 70-80 percent of your maximum. This is enough to push your muscles to become stronger. Yet you will keep within your ability. For safety, you should start at a level that is considerably low, at about 50-60%, to minimize the risk of injury.

Since you use muscles in daily life, it is easy to approximate your current strength. For example, if you often lift heavy objects – including your grandchildren – you might be a little bit stronger. If you walk every day, and take the stairs, your aerobic capacity might be better than that of a sedentary person.

Muscle Soreness

Because your body is not used to lifting weights, your muscles go through a greater degree of stress. So don't be surprise that you may feel pain during the first few weeks of training, but learn to identify helpful pain from serious injury.

In the first week you may feel fine, and then ache the next day. This is delayed muscle soreness. This soreness is typically mild and fades within two days. A hot bath can help to relax.

A bad pain is sharp and a signal to stop. It is not always a sign of injury, but a pre-existing joint problem. Nonetheless, stop the exercise. If the pain does not go away, but gets progressively more severe, seek medical attention.

During the next training try again, but be careful. Use lighter weights and limit the range of motion.

After twelve weeks, you will have gained significantly in strength. After six months, progress usually slows down as the body gets used to the exercises. You might want to try increasing the weights and repetitions. Sometimes, it's better to just enjoy your workout and keep at that level until the program becomes a habit. This is what you're working towards; to make this workout something automatic. Indeed, you may find that if you miss a few sessions, your body actually craves the exercise.

Chapter 8

ADDING AEROBIC
EXERCISES

For all of the health benefits of strength training, it doesn't train your heart and lungs. For that you need aerobic activity. Aerobics not only change your quality of life, they help extend it, including:

Improving the health of the lungs and cardiovascular
system.
Helping to tone muscles.
Losing weight (since they consume calories, it helps
burn fat.)
Providing emotional benefit by boosting self-esteem
and relieving depression, anxiety, stress and
insomnia.

Should I do aerobic exercise too?

No matter how busy you are, your heart deserves 30 minutes of your time. It doesn't have to be a solid block of time; three ten-minute sessions will do. Moderate exercise does not necessarily mean sports or the gym. Any activity that raises your heart rate counts. It's unfortunate but true: The more unfit you are, the less fun it is to exercise. Who wants to take a walk if your legs ache after five minutes? This is where strength training makes a big difference.

Advanced Exercises

These additional exercises can supplement your basic program. These new practices target important muscle groups in the upper and lower back the abdomen and the shoulders.

Trim and Flatten your Abdomen

Excess fat in the abdomen is associated with greater health risks for women than excess fat in the thighs and buttocks. The solution requires a combination of strength training to tone the abdominal muscles plus aerobic exercise.

These exercises strengthen your shoulders and back, increasing their range of motion

Abdominal Curl. Level 1

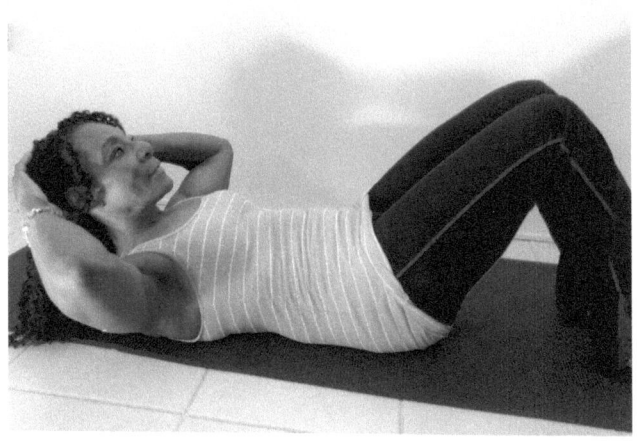

Lay on your back, making certain your head isn't too far forward, with your knees bent and your feet flat on the floor. Place your hands behind your ears at the base of your skull to support your head and lift your shoulders from the floor. Repeat 8 to 10 times.

Abdominal Curl. Level 2 (side)

Lay on your back with the knees bent and your feet flat on the floor. Your heels should be 6-8 cm from your buttocks. Place your hands behind your ears at the base of your skull to support your head and neck. Your eyes should be focused on the ceiling.

You will feel the effort in the centre of your abdomen and on both sides along your ribs. You should not feel a strain in your neck. Pay close attention to the position of your head and neck during the upward movement and concentrate on lifting only your shoulders off the ground. Repeat 8 to 10 times.

Pelvic Tilt:

This exercise is a classic; and for good reason. It trims and strengthens your entire midsection, buttocks, thighs, abdomen and back.

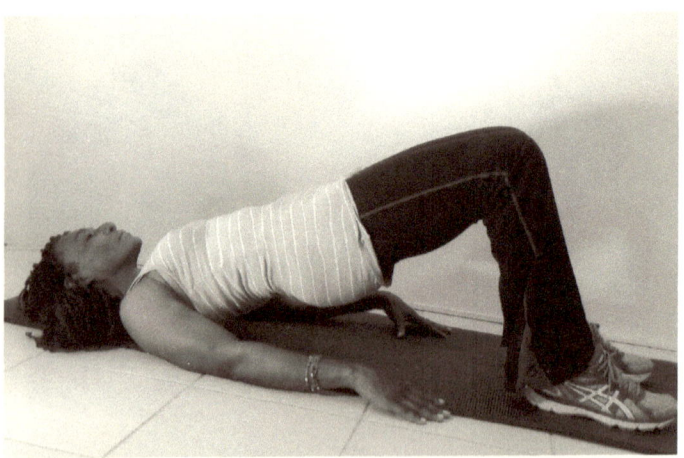

Lay on your back with the knees bent and your feet flat on the floor, shoulder-width apart. Your arms should be at your sides, palms flat. Roll your pelvis off the floor, keeping your midsection straight.

Push-Up

Push-ups are terrific but difficult for many women, since it requires strength in the upper body and muscles of the abdomen and back. And because you are using your bodyweight for resistance, push-ups don't require equipment.

Most women cannot do push-ups. The problem is not anatomy but information. Few women know how to do push-ups correctly. You may have to skip them, if you are suffering from serious knee, shoulder or back problems. As with any exercise, pain is a signal to be careful. It is important to do push-ups properly and that requires an amount of abdominal and back strength. So if you are able to do the push-ups, make sure to include the back and abdominal exercises as well.

Keep your elbow from locking move your shoulder just about over your hand, you can cross your knee to take the pressure off them.

Modified Level 1

Begin with the the modified push-up. When they become easier, move to level 2. Try to do as many as you can. Even if it is difficult in the beginning, don't give up. It gets easier with time. Make sure your palms are in place with your shoulders.

Push-Up Level 2

Begin in the same position as the level 1 modified push-up. As you push away from the floor, breathe out. Many people tend to hold their breath when doing this exercise. keep your neck and head in a straight line.

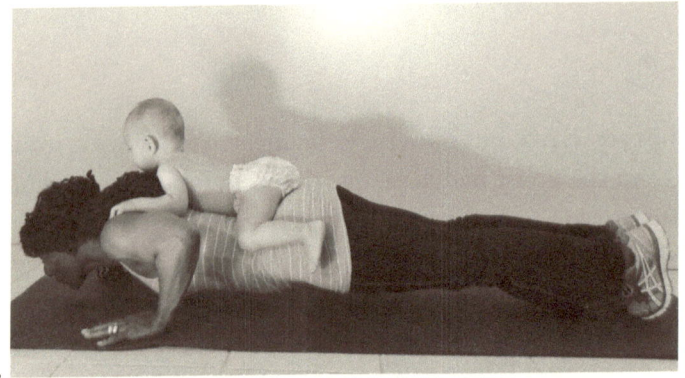

A.

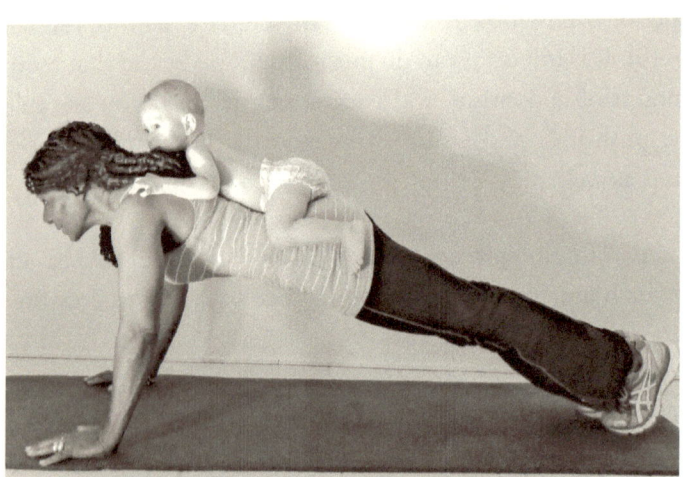

B.

Side Arm Raise (with dumbbells)

This movement may takes a little practice to master since the shoulder muscles of most women are weak. It may be better to start with no more than 1 or 2 kg. If you are under age fifty, you should eventually reach 4 to 6 kg. If you are over fifty, 3 to 4 kg.

When doing this movement, keep your elbows slightly bent. Don't scrunch your shoulder. You can sit on a chair or stand.

Bend your elbow and slowly lift your arms out to the side.

This exercise has a nice side benefit. When you wear a jacket with shoulder pads, it makes your waist and hips look smaller. The same thing happens when you build your shoulder muscles. Our bones are wider at the hips, but narrow around the shoulders. That's why we sometimes think we have big hips. Adding some muscle around the shoulders balances things out!

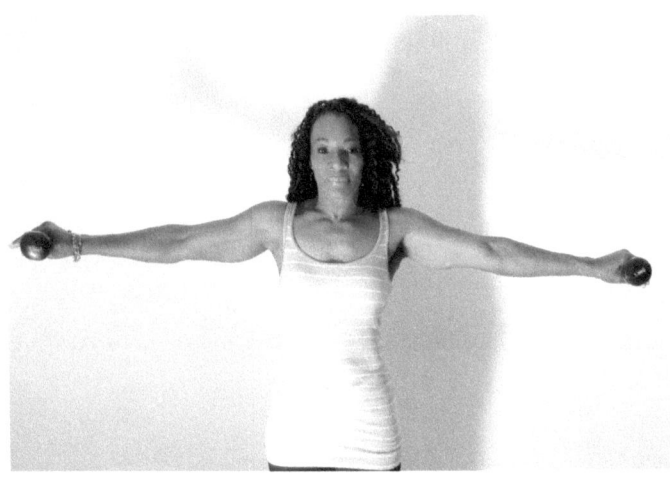

Lunge

If you have knee problems, be very careful when doing this exercise.

The lunge promotes strength coordination, balance and power. It help tightens your lower body and strengthens your lower back. There are two levels of the Lunge. Start with level 1. Keeping your feet shoulder-width apart, step forward. You may rely on a chair or wall for support in the beginning .

Lunge Level 2 can be with or without weights. The foot position is the same as level 1. If you still can not do it without holding on, then try one leg at a time for 8 to 10 repetitions. Remember to keep your your knees off the floor. The leading knee should not go past your toes.

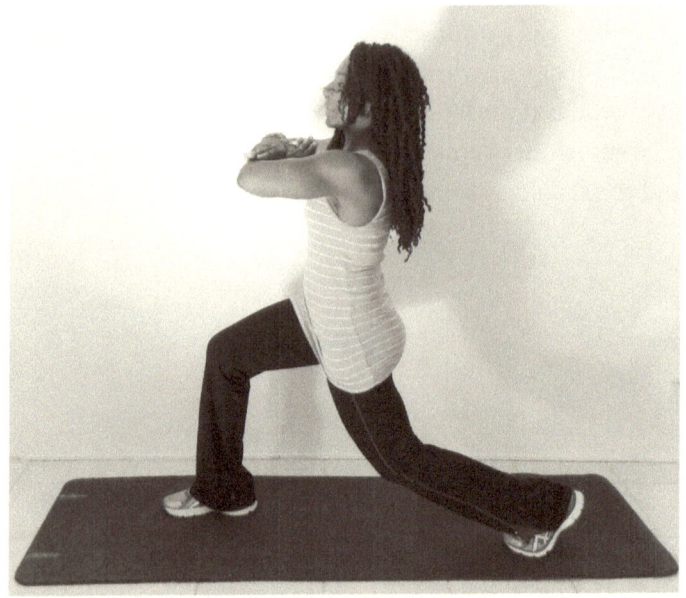

Chapter 11

GYM WORKOUTS

This is for women who want to workout at home while doing a strength training program. However, I will also give some ideas for the fitness studio. Things have changed over the past few years. Trainers have begun to understand the importance of a strength program.

It may be safer and less time consuming to do only cardio machines, but most gym weight-training workouts last about 45 minutes. There maybe more benefit using machines if you are new to fitness because machines can be controlled more easily to isolate your muscles, and you are also able to keep your body in the right position for the movement.

Knee Extension Machine

Adjust the backrest, so your knees are just over the edge of the seat. The centre of your knee joint should be in-line with the joint of the machine. This movement should be done slowly for 8 to 10 repetitions.

If you have knee problems, you can train one leg at a time. You may need to adjust the resistance of each leg.

Overhead Press

The seat height should be the same level as your shoulders, and your back firmly against the backrest. Raise your arms move over head until they are extended, 8 - 10 times.

Double Leg Press

A great exercise for buttocks and legs.

Caution: If possible, don't use a double leg press machine that positions you lying down with your shoulders against pads. This position puts a lot of pressure on the spine and shoulders.

Front Lateral Pull-Down

Pull-downs help the back from slumping. Lateral pull-downs also strengthen the bones in the spine (though women who are already very fit can use a chin-up bar at home).

Place your hands slightly wider than your shoulder-width. Lean back slightly from the hips so that the bar is slightly over your chest. Lift your chest and squeeze your shoulder blades together. Don't lock your elbows.

Leg Curl

The seated version of this machine is best, as it keep the stress off your lower back.

Adjust the backrest so that your knees are just over the edge of the seat. Your knee joints should align with the joint of the machine.

Biceps Curl

This exercise corresponds to the biceps curl done with dumbbells in the at-home version.

Make sure the joint on the arm of the machine is in line with your elbow joints. Repeat this 8-10 times.

Seated Row

Seated rowing is good for the lower and middle back. If you spend most of your day sitting in a chair, this exercise strengthens and improves your posture.

Keeping your arms parallel to the floor, bend forward while keeping the lower back straight. Repeat 8 - 10 times.

Back Extension

For a good posture that makes you look younger, slimmer and more confident. The back extension strengthens the lower back.

Cross your hands in-front of your chest. Slowly extend your body, keeping your chin slightly tipped to your chest. Repeat 8 - 10 times.

Abdominal Curl

Training the abdominal muscles stabilizes and protects your spine.

Lift your shoulder off the floor slowly as high as you can and return to the starting position. Repeat 8 - 10 times.

Toe Stand

This exercise is also used in the home program.

Men Need Strength Training, Too!

Men typically have more muscles and stronger bones than women. But they also lose strength, bone mass and balance as they get older. Beginning around age 30, men lose about 1 percent of their muscle strength annually. After 60, it accelerates to about 2 percent. By the time a man reaches his eightieth birthday, he typically loses about 60 percent of the strength he had at age 30.

Thanks to their head start, men take longer to reach the danger point. But if they live long enough, they too are at risk of falls and fractures. Fortunately, strength training can help. Men benefit in the same ways as women do.

The exercises in this book work just as well for men as they do for women. The only difference is that men can start with weights that are one or two kg heavier and they can expect to reach higher goals.

Questions & Answers

Q. Can this program help me lose weight?

A. Yes. Strength training – along with cutting calories and doing aerobic exercises – is an ideal way to lose fat. The more muscles you have, the higher your metabolic rate. This means that when you add strength training to your weight-loss program, you can eat more. Also, if you have been dieting and reached a plateau, strength training might help you move past this point.

Q. Can I do this program if I am pregnant?

A. I hope you will be inspired to become – or remain – active while you are pregnant to help prepare for birth. But I don't recommend that you begin with this program.

Q. I walk nearly an hour a day. Isn't that enough?

A. Walking is an excellent exercise. Like other aerobic activities, it increases longevity and decreases your risk of chronic diseases – but it is not enough. Walking doesn't benefit the hipbones. Strength training helps both the spine and hips.

Q. I sit at a desk all day and tend to lean forwards. Will strength training help me?

A. Women who sit at work often have poor posture and back problems – as do those whose jobs keep them on their feet but not moving. Exercises that strengthen the shoulders and upper back will help.

Q. Will strength training affect how well I do other sports?

A. Yes – and it will reduce the risk of injury too. That's why competitive athletes add strength-training exercises to their regimes. If you are active in a particular sport, be aware that some of your muscles may be very well conditioned while others are not. For instance, a runner may have well developed legs, but undeveloped arms. A tennis player's racket arm may be muscular while the other is not. So a program that improves overall fitness will be helpful.

Q. Can I follow this program if I have a bad back?

A. Talk to your physician first. Most people with back problems can do this program and benefit from it. Start at the beginning level and work up slowly. Concentrate on maintaining good posture.

Q. I have osteoporosis. Is strength training safe for me?

A. This program is also for people with osteoporosis condition. It is not only safe, but beneficial. It is important to check with your doctor first, because you may have special needs. Start the basic program with one-kilo weights and progress slowly, increasing the weight as you grow stronger. Your bones will get as strong as your muscles but they need more time. Talk to your doctor if you want to add exercises for the back and the abdomen.

Q. I have arthritis. How will this affect my strength training?

A. Don't exercise a joint that under an arthritis attack. Wait a few days. If you have difficulty holding the hand weights, use wrist weights instead. Progress slowly.

Q. I have diabetes. Will this affect strength training?

A. Studies have shown that strength training has particular benefits for people with diabetes. If you have diabetes, discuss strength training with your doctor before you begin. As with any new exercise, you will need to monitor your glucose level closely. Remember to breathe properly when you lift to avoid increasing vascular pressure.

Q. I am extremely busy during the week. Can't I do two sessions on Saturday and Sunday?

A. I don't recommend this. To gain the maximum benefit, you need a day between workouts so your muscles have time to repair themselves. You can break the session into two parts, arms one day and legs the other day.

Q. How long should I wait after eating before doing exercises?

A. It is best to wait until you are no longer full, usually an hour or more.

Q. I want to do aerobics and strength training – how do I combine them?

A. The usual recommendation for aerobics is to work out for 30 minutes three to six days a week. You can add a complete strength training program to your workout two or three of those days or a few exercises every day so long as you don't work the same muscles two days in a row. You can do aerobics first to warm up, then strength training.

Q. I have been doing strength training for some months and now feel a pain in my hip joints when doing the side hip raises.

A. If you are experiencing pain from the exercises, it is clear that you should have your hip checked. Discontinue exercises that give you pain. A mild ache is normal in the beginning; but you should not experience acute pain or discomfort with the exercise.

Q. I have been following the program for a while and seem to have reached my limit. What do I do now for maintenance?

A. Keep strength training twice a week. You needn't increase the weights, but I suggest you change exercises periodically. You will work more muscles, and your program will remain fresh.

You've Taken Care of Your Muscles:
But Don't Forget Your Skin!

Just as rings show the age of a tree, wrinkles show the age of a person. Your skin tells your story. Be nice to it. Here are the basic principles of skin care:

Cleanse your face twice a day, in the morning and at bedtime.

Drink plenty of water to moisturize it from the inside.

Get enough sleep. Lack of sleep invites dark circles and a pallor that can make you look older.

Drink alcohol in moderation.

Eat a balanced diet of protein, vegetables, salads and fruits

A bit of sun is okay. But too much is your skin's worst enemy!

PART 3

NUTRITION

Chapter 12

NUTRITION OVERVIEW

It's a horrible fact, but one that needs to be faced: as we age, our diets must change. The same diet you had in your twenties is likely to wreak havoc on you in your fifties.

I personally have tried every trick on how to eat and what vitamins and supplements to take. Even my exercises I had to change.

I first became interested in nutrition after my first world championship. I noticed that most of my US competitors were always ahead of me. Having heard from one of them about their nutrition plan, I decided to take some courses in nutrition. At the time, the instructors gave little emphasis to the missing connection between sports and nutrition. I began asking questions, reading what information I could and changed my eating habits. Although most nutritionists I talked to were tied into particular dietary schools of thought, they were similar to conventional physicians, who will only prescribe conventional treatments. Alternative practitioners do the same. Nutritionists are specialists in certain diets and recommend these diets to their clients. They can give you only the knowledge they have; this may or may not be the best for you. This is not a criticism, but a fact that will help you make the best decision.

To be successful, you do not need to become a nutritionist yourself. You need to identify how you feel, how your body reacts to the food you eat, You need to widen your knowledge of nutrition to be in the position to determine what food is right for you. To reach this goal you need to forget the old food pyramid, throw away your diet books and spend some time understanding how food affects your hormone balance. More importantly, avoid unhealthy eating habits such as:

> Too much Alcohol.
> Soda (sugar free and regular.)
> Chocolate.
> Ice cream.
> Desserts.
> Too much pasta, pizza, starch and bread.
> Eating late at night or not eating enough.

Tina's Words of Wisdom: Put the scale away!

If you are one of those people that go on the scale every morning, it seems to control your life. There are 6.2 billion people on the planet; no two persons are exactly the same. Just as people are born with different eyes, hair and skin colour, people inherit different metabolic processes, influencing the building of muscle and fat loss. Some people have genetics that make it difficult to lose body fat. For those people, informed food choices are essential for a long life.

How many times have you heard that fruits have too much sugar, grains have too much starch, meat is acid-forming or that nuts are too high in fat? This obsessing is far more toxic than the foods themselves!

Of course, there are things I eat rarely; others, I don't eat at all. I avoid milk and dairy products. These are choices each of you have to make for yourself. Be aware of the subconscious guilt causing less enjoyable eating, however. Regard your body as a temple and your food as an offering to it. See your meals as loving gifts to yourself. You are not eating to harm yourself or adhere to a system or impress anybody. You are eating to get stronger and feel younger.

Chapter 13

FROM THE PYRAMID
TO THE PLATE

If you are a member of the baby boomer generation, you probably grew up believing that the food pyramid was an ideal guide for proper nutrition. But things have changed. On June 2, 2011, Michelle Obama unveiled the new, USDA-approved MyPlate model. The food pyramid focused on animal products and processed foods, as opposed to whole plant foods. Here are some of the changes featured:

> Balancing calories as opposed to counting calorie. This means you can enjoy your food, but try to eat less and avoid oversize portions.
> Make half your plate fruits and vegetables.
> Make at least half your grains whole grains.
> Switch from milk to water and fresh vegetables or fruit juice. Dairy plays a less significant role than it did in the original food pyramid.
> Choose low sodium foods. Sodium can raise your blood pressure and makes you retain water.
> Drink water instead of sugary drinks.

> Protein is now a general category, whereas the old pyramid specified meats, fish and poultry as proteins. MyPlate gives you the option of choosing other protein sources.

A side note on lactose intolerance:

Are you having trouble flattening your belly? It might be lactose intolerance. The results of a study performed at John Hopkins University show that 75 percent of African-American, Jewish, Latino and Native American adults are lactose intolerant, while some 90 percent of Asian-Americans are lactose intolerant. Stomach bloat followed by pain is one symptom. If you are lactose intolerant, you can get calcium from green vegetables, such as collard greens, turnip greens, broccoli, and kale.

Chapter 14

ALL ABOUT WATER

Without water, there is no fat loss. Unfortunately, most people don't drink enough of it. Despite this resource all around us, and flowing through us, people still remain unaware of the role that water plays in our body chemistry. Approximately 60-70% of the human body is composed of water. Blood is 90% water, muscles are 70% and bones retain roughly 20% water.

Water works like a regulator for body temperature. Nutrients that build tissues, lubricate joints and expedite digestion and circulation depend on water as the pathway by which they function.

I am often told water has no taste. But, it doesn't need to. Try drinking a glass of water each time you crave unhealthy food. You need six to eight glasses of water each day. Coffee, cola and even black tea with antioxidants contain caffeine, a diuretic that triggers dehydration. Instead, choose mineral water, caffeine free herbal teas, juice or fresh fruits and vegetables. An apple contains 66 percent water, raw cauliflower 82 percent. Cantaloupe or uncooked spinach is 84 percent water.

People who eat large amounts and salad and fresh fruit can drink fewer glasses of water than those who do not.

Tool 21: Drink From the
Fountain of Youth

You can't talk about nutrition without talking about water. Water is the primary ingredient of the fountain of youth.

If you want every organ inside you to work properly, you need water. If you want your kidneys to work throughout your life, you need water. If you want great skin and bright eyes, you need water. Almost every chemical reaction in your body needs water. Every molecule in your body needs water. Without it, your cells go on strike and refuse to act.

Chapter 15

VITAMINS AND DIETARY SUPPLEMENTS

The amount of vitamins and supplements on the market are simply overwhelming. But after thirty years of taking vitamins and supplement, I've seen definitive results. This list of supplements will correctly enhance hormone balance and help keep you healthy. Your decisions here may be adjusted according to age and needs. Consult a physician or nutritional expert before adding them to your plan.

- Vitamin C
- L. Carnitine
- Coenzyme Q10
- Omega 3 DHA
- Calcium, magnesium and zinc
- L -Glutamine

Vitamin C

Vitamin C is undisputed as a premier antioxidant. It can help clean up toxins created by every cell in the body. Vitamin C is involved in practically every chemical process in our body. It is indirectly involved in the manufacturing of hormones, in the production of blood cells and immune system enhancement. Even though you might eat lots of citrus and green vegetables, many people still have a deficit of Vitamin C.

L -Carnitine

L-Carnitine is an amino acid found in meat. It is not an essential amino acid but a critical one, a building block for proteins and hormones. Studies have proven that L-Carnitine is an important substrate for hormone production and a critical factor in the process of energy production at the cellular level, as well as for moving fatty acids and helping with the production of energy. In every cell that contains L-Carnitine, hormones are produced.

Coenzyme Q10

Coenzyme Q10 is found in every cell in the human body. Q10 is also an important partner to the working of L-Carnitine in the process of energy production. It is a stronger antioxidant than vitamin E. New research into the cardio-protective capabilities of Q10 has helped increase its popularity in recent years.

Omega 3 Fatty Acids

Found in fish-oil, this nutrient eases inflammation, particularly as a result of joint disease and has been proven to help lower cholesterol.

Vitamin B Complex or multivitamins

Usually include the following:

Vitamin B1 - Thiamine

Thiamine is a water soluble vitamin, which is necessary for metabolizing protein, carbohydrates and fats. It is also involved in the energy production cycle along with Coenzyme Q10.

Vitamin B5 - Pantothenic Acid

Pantothenic Acid is a water soluble B-vitamin. It is also involved in the processes of energy production and hormone formation. Deficiency can be associated with fatigue, depression and sleep disturbance.

Vitamin B6 - Pyridoxine

The most important function of B-6 is being part of the chemical reaction involving amino acids, leading to the production of hormones. Studies show it enhances brain function and sleep.

Vitamin B12 - Cyanocobalamin

Vitamin B12 is directly involved in the chemical processes that lead to hormone production and maintenance, as well as enhancing brain function and sleep.

Calcium

Calcium has an essential role in keeping our hearts regular and balancing the production of stomach and pancreatic enzymes. Necessary for proper food digestion and absorption, calcium can be found in dairy products like milk, cheese and green leafy vegetables like broccoli and spinach.

Magnesium

Working in conjunction with calcium, magnesium is directly involved in hundreds of chemical reactions taking place in our body; from maintenance of the immune system to energy production. It is found naturally in many foods, including whole grain products, fruits and vegetables, meat, poultry and fish.

Zinc

Zinc plays an important role in the synthesis of protein and fat. It also helps with alcohol metabolism, insulin function and protection of the immune system. It can be found in meat, dairy, soy and whole grain products.

L-Glutamine

L-Glutamine is stored primarily in muscle cells. It prevents insulin spikes through a mechanism of balance in blood sugar levels. L-Glutamine is present in beans, fish, meat and dairy products.

Colostrum

Colostrum is the first mother's milk, protecting newborn babies from viral infections, allergies and toxins. Derived from dairy cows, it is taken to enhance immunity. To keep your body and immune globulin intact, use it off and on as a supplement to your diet.

Tips on Preventing Osteoporosis

Building and maintaining healthy bones is a life-long investment. The sooner you start the better. The most important measures are:

1) Make sure you get enough calcium and Vitamin D. Take supplements if necessary.
2) Do strengthening exercises to build bone.
3) Discuss bone density with your doctor if you are at risk.

Recommended Calcium-rich Foods

Soy milk	8 ounces	200 – 300 mgs
Spinach	½ cup	125 mg

Other leafy greens, bok choy

Cabbage, all cooked	½ cup	50 mg
Leafy greens, raw	1 cup	50 mg
Beans, cooked	1 cup	50 - 120 mgs
Salmon (canned with bones)	3 ounces	200 mg
Rhubarb	½ cup	175 mg
Tofu	½ cup	250 mg
Yoghurt	8 ounces	275 – 325 mgs

Chapter 16

UNDERSTANDING BODY FAT AND HOW IT WORKS

Goodness me, "I am getting fatter". Welcome to menopause!

Body fat is the most confusing aspect of dieting and exercise for most people to understand. My students don't understand it. Neither do some dieticians. It took me 20 years of research to tap into the mystery of body fat. This book is based on a combination of scientific information, combined with my own experience throughout my competition years. The recommendations I make are for losing body fat, without compromising good health. But first you must understand the biochemistry of fat.

Our diet has changed dramatically over the past century. There was a time when we ate natural foods that were made without the use of chemicals or added flavours. Now, packaged foods – high in pesticides, chemicals, and refined sugars – fill the grocery aisles.

Doctors and nutritionists eagerly weigh in with theories about the consequences of these changes. They blame everything from cancer to obesity on these changes. What we don't get is how subtle dietary changes impact our health and our environment.

Tool 22: The story behind the Omegas

Omega-6 fatty acids belong to the essential fatty acid family. Your body needs them, but it can't make them. Subsequently, they have to come from food. Omega-6 fatty acids collaborate with omega-3 fatty acids to help maintain brain function. They also stimulate skin and hair growth, maintain bone density and regulate metabolism. These are important factors for women of a certain age.

A healthy diet balances omega-3 and omega-6 fatty acids. Omega-3 fatty acids help reduce inflammation, while some omega-6 fatty acids tend to promote inflammation. Diets in the United States usually contain 20 - 25 times more omega-6 fatty acids than omega-3 fatty acids.

Anthropological studies tell us that our hunter-gatherer ancestors ate omega-6 and omega-3 fats in a one to one ratio. The results of these studies also indicate that modern inflammatory diseases, such as heart disease, cancer, and diabetes, were conspicuous in their absence among our ancestors.

In contrast, the Mediterranean diet has a healthier balance between omega-3 and omega-6 fatty acids. This diet is low in meat products (which are high in omega-6 fatty acids) but consists of rich foods which contains lots of omega-3 fatty acids like whole grains, fresh fruits and vegetables, fish, olive oil and garlic. A moderate amount of wine can complement any diet.

White flour, meat and other animal products as well as cooking oil other than olive and canola are omega-6 sources. Sources of omega-3 are cold-water fish like salmon, cod, trout and mackerel, English walnuts and flax seeds or oil. You can also take supplementary EFAs in capsule form (fish oil or for vegetarians EFAs that are algae derived). EFAs deteriorate very rapidly and are sensitive to light and oxygen as well as heat. Too much exposure to any of these changes the oil's molecular structure from natural and health-promoting to damaging and toxic.

Chapter 17

ABOUT FAT BURNING

Dieting confuses your body. Especially extreme dieting. During crash diets, your body feeds off itself, burning fat stores, muscles and even internal organs for energy. Unfortunately, this life preserving mechanism can work against you when you are trying to lose body fat, because your body cannot tell the difference between dieting and starvation. The consequences of a low calorie diet are automatic and unavoidable; the responses are metabolic and hormonal. It responds with decreased metabolism, loss of muscle, and increased activity of fat-storing enzymes and hormones.

It's interesting to note the same thing happens during dehydration. When you don't drink enough water, your belly bloats. Just as extra fat storage keeps you alive during starvation diets, bloat protects you from dehydration. So losing weight is not about taking extreme measures: It's about forming new habits.

The first step to losing body fat permanently has more to do with your mind than it does with nutrition or exercise. You have to change your entire attitude about nutrition and exercise. Instead of thinking of diet, adopt the mindset of a lifelong habits. Once a habit is firmly established, it takes enormous strength to break it.

To lose body fat you must maintain a negative caloric balance. This might entail decreasing caloric intake, increasing energy expenditure or a combination of the two. For example, if you are a woman with a maintenance level of 2100 calories per day, then a deficit of 500 puts you at 1600 calories per day.

A 500-calorie deficit over seven days works out to 3500 calories in one week. There are over 7000 calories in a kilo of fat, resulting in a loss of a 1/2 kilo per week. Fat loss seldom follows these calculations precisely. An emphasis on exercise with a small reduction in calories is the best way to lose body fat. A 500 to 750 calorie deficit below your maintenance level is usually plenty. Add your weight training and aerobics. Remember: to lose body weight there must be a calorie deficit. However, there is more than one way to create a calorie deficit. One way is to decrease your calorie intake from food; the other is to increase the amount of calories you burn through exercise.

There are some reasons why exercise is a better method of burning fat than dieting. One is that exercise, in particular strength training and aerobics, raises your metabolic rate, creating a calorie deficit without triggering the starvation response. It literally signals to your body to keep your muscles and not burn them for energy. Dieting without exercise can result in up to 50% of the weight loss from muscles themselves. Exercise also increases fat-burning enzymes and hormones. Finally, exercise increases your cell's sensitivity to insulin so that carbohydrates are burned for energy and stored as glycogen rather than fat.

The best way to lose body fat permanently without losing muscles is to lose weight slowly with the focus on exercise rather than severe calorie cutting.

Losing more than 1 kilo per week means you should actually eat more! I know this may be difficult for you when you want to lose fat. But if you lose more than the recommended amount you are not only losing fat but muscles, too!

Tool 23: Building muscle burns fat

Muscle is your weapon against fat. Muscle is active tissue, a fast acting catalyst for your metabolism. Although watching TV is non active, your muscles are still burning calories. Fat, in comparison, simply sits there wasting energy.

Chapter 18

THE COMPLEXITY
OF CALORIES

As I mentioned earlier, there are 6.2 billion people on the planet and no two people are the same. People with a genetic disposition to weight gain have an uphill challenge losing body fat and have to make smart food choices. This is essential to living a long and healthy life. Nonetheless, obsessing about food causes stress, and actually speeds up the aging process.

As I said, your body is a temple; your food, an offering. You are not eating to impress anybody. You are eating to get stronger and feel younger. While eating with others can be a joy, it also can be challenging. You may notice some people may not be supportive of your changes. If possible, avoid those people until you can stand on your own without stressing yourself. Learning to analyze calorie intake can be a healthy aspects of controlling your amount of food. It should not destroy the joy of eating. If you don't enjoy the experience, you may find yourself raiding the refrigerator when you get home.

Understanding Calories

Definition of a calorie

There is a lot of talk about calories yet many people still do not really understand the technical definition. Simply, let's just say it's the amount of heat required to raise one kilo (1 liter) of water 1 C°. A calorie is simply a measurement of heat energy. To draw an analogy, body fat is like reserve storage for energy. Burning body fat is nothing more than releasing calories from your "storage tank" during activities. If you are inactive, the fat stays in the tank until you need it. Your energy reserves are still serving as an important purpose. In our society, where famine is not the same concern in western countries as it was for our ancestors, body fat is more of a cosmetic problem or health risk.

From this basic understanding, you should recognize the importance of counting calories and keeping track of the amount of food you eat. Your intake of calories is just as important as keeping track of your bank account. If you fail to pay attention to your withdrawals, you would soon find yourself in debt. It's the same with your body.

Despite the obvious importance of watching your intake, there are many diet programs insisting you can eat anything if you eat the right "secret" combination of foods. In our lazy and pleasure-seeking society this idea sounds wonderful; but physiologically, it's impossible.

To complicate matters, caloric requirement varies among people with similar activity levels. If you want to be slim, choose your parents wisely! In other words, we inherit our metabolic rates from mom and dad. Joking aside, it does not mean if your parents are overweight, you have to be. It just means you have inherited BMR, or Basal Metabolic Rate. BMR is the total number of calories your body burns for normal bodily function like digestion, circulation and respiration, but not including physical exertion. Knowing your heredity will help you understand what you need to do. You do not have to be overweight if your parents are; it just means you will have to live a more active and calorie conscious lifestyle.

How To Determine Your Daily Calorie Maintenance

Once you understand the importance of calories the first step in finding out your personal fat loss plan is to calculate the total number of calories you burn every day, or your total daily energy expenditure (DEE.) This is the level where your calorie deposits are equal to your calorie withdrawals, meaning the amount of calories your body burns within 24 hours.

According to many exercise physiologists, the average female maintenance level is around 2000-2100 calories per day. The actual calorie use is higher for athletes or extremely active people. Calorie requirement can also vary among people with the same activity levels because of differences in inherited metabolic rates.

Your total body weight and body size are major factors for the number of calories you need. The bigger you are, the more calories you will require.

The higher your Lean Body Mass (i.e. muscle) the higher your BMR will be. Muscle is active tissue and it requires much energy to maintain it. That's why weight training helps you lose body fat.

Men usually require more calories than women. The average inactive male has a maintenance level of 2000-2100 calories per day. The average inactive woman has 1500-2000 calories per day.

A fast and easy way to determine how many calories you need is to use your current body weight times 24. To lose weight without activity reduce your calories by 15-20% below maintenance level.

The higher your body mass, the higher your BMR (Basal Metabolic Rate.) This is important if you want to lose body fat, because lean mass plays a role. The more muscle you have, the more calories you will burn at rest. The best way to increase your BMR is to increase your LBM. This is why weight training is important in losing body fat.

Although it may not be necessary to write down the amount of calories you eat every day for the rest of your life, it is important you take control over your eating habit. If you want to keep your weight in balance you must understand how calories work.

Eating small, frequent meals helps prevent you from overeating through portion control. Excess calories at one meal will always be converted into body fat.

Eating time:

Ideally you should begin eating early, so you can eat five to six meals a day. It is best to consume the last meal two to three hours before going to bed. On average, the optimal calorie intake per day for women is somewhere between 1500-1600. As you get older, you will need less food. To get your ideal calorie intake per meal is easy; just divide your daily calorie intake by the number of meals you eat. For example, the optimal caloric intake for fat loss is 1500. If the number of of meals is 5, then your calorie intake per meal should be 300.

This is a better solution than skipping meals. When you skip meals your body's need for amino acids does not stop. When you cut off continual flow of amino acids from protein, it simply takes it from your own muscle. Starving yourself to lose weight or even missing meals puts you in a catabolic state; you literally eat your own muscle tissue. Your body does not store protein. Amino acids only remain in your bloodstream for about three hours. This is why it's important to eat every few hours.

For a short period of time, when maximum fat loss is desired, you should eat 50-55% carbohydrates; 30% protein and 15-20% fat. This increases the metabolism through the thermal effect of food and controls the insulin more effectively.

Reducing carbohydrates and increasing protein can give you some hormonal and metabolic advantages when it comes to fat loss.

A high protein/low carbohydrate diet will cause quicker fat loss,but you'll also experience a decrease of energy, a loss of muscle and slow down your metabolism. The more you reduce your carbohydrates, the greater the side effects and the more difficult it will be to maintain your fat loss after you have reached your goal.

> 1 gram of carbohydrate = 4 calories
> 1 gram of protein = 4 calories
> 1 gram of fat = 9 calories.

Chapter 19

WHY PROTEIN?

Your body is constantly creating new cells. These come from food, specifically protein. Protein is the raw construction material for body cells. Structures made from protein include skin, hair, nails, and bones and of course muscle. Protein is critical for the body. It makes up about 15-20% of body weight.

As much talk as there is about carbohydrates, the knowledge of protein is still in the dark ages. Women still think if they eat protein they'll develop huge muscles like a bodybuilder. Speaking as a former professional one, it took me 6 hours a day, 5 days a week of heavy training training to develop even a little bulk muscle.

Animal protein sources include animal meat, fish and dairy products; including milk, cheese, yoghurt, buttermilk, eggs and sour cream.

Nitrogen Balance

Fats, proteins and carbohydrates are also composed of carbon, hydrogen and oxygen, but only protein can bring nitrogen into the body. If the intake of nitrogen is more than the amount excreted, protein is being retained and muscle is being built. If more nitrogen is excreted than is consumed, you have a negative nitrogen balance; meaning protein is being broken down and muscle is being lost.

The smallest units of a protein are called amino acids. These are the building blocks of protein. There are 20 amino acids required for growth by the human body. From these, there are tens of thousands of different protein molecules. Each is assembled from the bonding of different amino acids into various configurations.

Out of the twenty amino acids, the body can produce eleven by itself, known as non-essential amino acids. The other nine are called essential amino acids and cannot be manufactured by your body; they must be supplied from food.

Protein is not wholly found in meat, fish and dairy. There are also proteins in vegetables, beans, legumes and grains.

Because protein cannot be stored for later use like carbohydrates, it is necessary to consume a complete protein in every meal to stay in a positive nitrogen balance. Your goal should be to include a source of complete protein with every meal and eat five to six small meals per day.

Complete lean proteins include:

Chicken breast, turkey, fish, shellfish, eggs (mostly whites – using limited yolks), lean red meat, low-fat dairy products, whey-based protein powders, soy, vegetables, beans and lentils.

Note: despite the popularity in eating high animal protein, it is harder for the body to digest.

About vegetarian diets

I became a vegetarian after 50 years of eating meat. This wasn't out of idealism; it was the only way to keep my body weight down. Going vegetarian made it a little more difficult to get the right amount of protein as it took more time to figure out my daily intake of protein, but there were no difficulties in building or keeping my muscles, and staying slim was easy. Vegetarians should include grains like quinoa, wild rice and garbanzo beans.

Some studies show that mortality from ischemic heart disease was 30% lower among vegetarian men and 20% lower among vegetarian women than in non-vegetarians. Vegetarian diets offer lower levels of saturated fat cholesterol, and higher levels of carbohydrates, fiber, magnesium, potassium and antioxidants such as vitamins C and E; as well as phytochemicals (non-nutritive plants chemicals that have disease preventative properties) Vegetarians also tend to have lower body mass index, lower levels of cholesterol, lower blood pressure, and less incidence of heart disease, hypertension type 2 diabetes and other disorders.

Some vegetable protein sources include beans, nuts, yams, soy and lentils.

What are carbohydrates?

There is a lot of talk these days about not eating carbohydrates. In fact, in many vegetarian restaurants I often see women leave carbohydrates untouched on their plates.

Unlike proteins, which are used as building material, carbohydrates are used for energy, particularly high intensity exercise. Carbohydrates are the body's most efficient energy source. Whenever they are restricted, energy levels and performance usually is low. Understanding how much you are using and what your daily need is is extremely important.

There are two broad categories of carbohydrates: simple and complex.

Simple carbohydrates are single sugar molecules including fructose. Glucose and fructose (fruit sugar) and (blood sugar) the biggest of all evil. Glucose is produced in the body through the breakdown of complex carbohydrates. Fructose is the type of simple carbohydrate found in fruit. There is a misunderstanding that to lose weight one should eat only fruits because they are healthier. But we are talking about keeping calories down, and there is just as much calories in sugar as in fact, and typically more harmful.

I remember when our daily carbohydrates came mostly from bread, because there was no other source. Today, I advise most of my clients to stop eating it due to the high glucose.

Simple carbohydrates

Eating too much causes blood sugar peaks. Your body responds to blood sugar peaks by releasing large amounts of insulin. The body overreacts, producing too much insulin, leading to a sharp drop in blood sugar. Low blood sugar is accompanied by craving, hunger, weakness, mood swings and a decrease in energy.

Complex carbohydrates

To lose body fat effectively, you should maintain a steady blood sugar level. This is where fibrous carbohydrates play a big role because they take longer to break down and digest than simple carbohydrates, which give a higher thermic effect,

There are two types of complex carbohydrates: starchy and fibrous. The difference is important to remember. Starch is the energy for the body, found in plants, potatoes, cereals, grains, bread, pasta, rice, oats, wheat and beans.

Fiber is the indigestible portion of the plant and therefore passes straight through your digestive tract without all the caloric energy being absorbed. Eating Fibrous carbohydrates for health benefits is important, but fiber also plays a major role in reducing body fat. The reason for this is that fibrous carbohydrates (such as green vegetables) contain very few calories and can be eating in great amount

Fiber rich foods include: apples, asparagus, berries, bok Choy, bran, broccoli, brussel sprouts, cabbage, cauliflower, cucumbers, eggplant, lettuce, oats, peas, peppers, radishes, spinach, string beans, turnips, watercress and zucchini.

So far we have talked about the difference between simple and complex carbohydrates, starchy and fibrous complex carbohydrates. If you don't understand yet, make it a habit to read labels and watch out for refined sugars. Most of the time you will find this information on the label.

The media industry has brainwashed people into believing that all fat is bad and the cause of obesity and health problems. Truth is, most fat-free products are almost 100% refined sugar. In fact, refined sugars and other highly processed foods are more responsible for poor health and obesity.

Fat and you

If the problem of obesity was solved, many people will be out of a job. As mad as it may sound, it's ultimately you who needs to take responsibility for your own health. There are far too many people who will be more than happy to make money off of you. When I started eating organic 30 years ago, only hippies were interested in pure food. Now, as the interest grows, so does the health industry. Healthy living has become a lifestyle which has opened the door to big money. And despite all the information about nutrition out there, there is still a great need for understanding how fat works in the body.

Fat is stored in the body as a backup energy source. Your body can also store carbohydrates, but in much more limited quantities. Carbohydrates are stored in your muscles and liver in the form of glycogen. About 400 grams of glycogen can be stored in the muscles (1600 calories) and about 100 grams (400 calories) in the liver.

Your body is always burning a mixture of carbohydrate and fat for fuel. During low intensity, long duration exercises, most of your energy comes from body fat. Most of your energy also comes from fat while you are at rest. During short bouts of high intensity exercise such as sprinting or weightlifting, the main fuel source is glycogen.

Your body can easily use fat for fuel. Even in lean people there is enough fat stored to last for a long time.

Final Words: Changing Old Habits, Learning New Routines

Changing habits is not easy, but must be done. If you have noticed any changes in the past 15 days after reading this book, you are well on the way to a connection between your body and your outlook. Maybe you've already started to eat differently. Perhaps by the time you've finished these words, you'll have adopted a healthier lifestyle. Congratulations! You are on your way to a fitter, healthier and more balanced you.

The next step takes place in your closet. Divide the clothes you own into two groups – the ones you really like and feel great wearing and the ones you put up with because they hide the fat. Divide them again into clothes you need and clothes you can get rid of. Consider this final tip a way of making room for a new life.

Be the person you really are, not the person people expect you to be.

Be willing to see things differently.

Believe in yourself and life will show the purpose for living.

Every situation has two sides.

Help others and they will help you.

Recognize that beauty is a feeling, not a number.

While you can't change everything, you can take responsibility for your own happiness.

Thanks to my daughters for letting me be the person I am today: Deborah, Brenda, Tamare and Sasha.

Also thank to Peter van Duyn who give me nothing but give me everything.